EMERGENCY ROPING AND BOULDERING

SURVIVAL ROPING, ROCK-CLIMBING, AND KNOT TYING

SAM FURY

Illustrated by
DIANA MANGOBA AND RAUL GUAJARDO

Copyright SF Nonfiction Books © 2017

www.SFNonfictionBooks.com

All Rights Reserved
No part of this document may be reproduced without written consent from the author.

WARNINGS AND DISCLAIMERS

The information in this publication is made public for reference only.

Neither the author, publisher, nor anyone else involved in the production of this publication is responsible for how the reader uses the information or the result of his/her actions.

CONTENTS

Introduction   vii

USEFUL KNOTS
Knot Tying Terms   3
10 Useful Knots   6

EMERGENCY ROPING
Descending   17
Ascending   19
Improvised Harnesses   24
Self-Rescue Bowline   26
River Crossing with Rope   28
Making a Gill Net   30
Making Rope   32
Throwing Rope   35

BOULDERING
Safety Tap   39
Basic Principles   41
Holds and Grips   43
Foot Techniques   49
Mantle   52
Types of Faces   57
Crack Climbing   59

References   63

Author Recommendations   65
About Sam Fury   67

THANKS FOR YOUR PURCHASE

Did you know you can get FREE chapters of any SF Nonfiction Book you want?

https://offers.SFNonfictionBooks.com/Free-Chapters

You will also be among the first to know of **FREE** review copies, discount offers, bonus content, and more.

Go to:

https://offers.SFNonfictionBooks.com/Free-Chapters

Thanks again for your support.

INTRODUCTION

This book is presented in three parts:

Knots

This section describes how to tie 10 knots that are described in other parts of this manual. These knots are also very useful in everyday life.

Emergency Roping

Emergency roping is the ability to use rope, without any other specialist equipment, to aid you in ascension and/or rappelling. It also covers the making of improvised rope and the use of rope for other aspects of survival.

Bouldering

Bouldering is climbing without the use of ropes or harnesses. It is also great for all-body toning and workout.

USEFUL KNOTS

Anyone can tie lots of knots, but a proper knot will be stronger and easier to untie.

There are many knots, far too many for the average person to remember. Fortunately, there is no need to remember them all. Just being able to tie a handful of knots is enough to see you through any situation when a knot is needed.

This section explains how to tie 10 knots that are discussed throughout the rest of this manual. They are also useful in everyday life.

These knots are from *The Useful Knots Book* by Sam Fury.

www.SurvivalFitnessPlan.com/Useful-Knots-Book

KNOT TYING TERMS

For ease of explanation when describing how to tie knots the following terminology will be used.

Bight

Any bend in-between the ends of the rope which does not cross over itself.

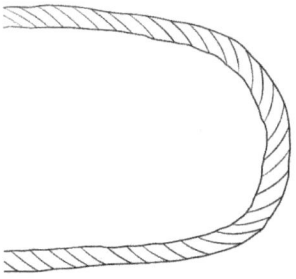

Crossing Point

The point where the rope crosses over itself.

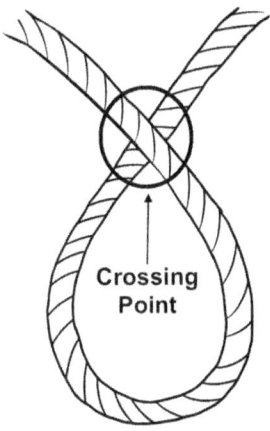

Load

Refers to the weight of the object being secured, e.g., if you are pulling a log then the log is the load.

Loop

Similar to a bight but the ends cross over, hence creating a closed circle.

An overhand loop is when the running end lies over the top of the standing part. An underhand loop is opposite (the standing part lies on top of the running end).

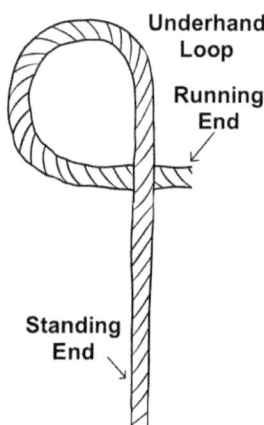

Rope

A generic term used in this book that refers to cord, rope, string, twine, or whatever material which is being used to tie a knot.

Running End

The part of the rope used to tie the knot. Also known as the working end.

Standing End

The part of the rope other than the running end.

Shock Load

Shock load occurs when there is a sudden increase in load. In such a case the load will be much more than the actual weight of the object. An example of this is when a climber falls and his/her weight suddenly loads the rope.

Turn

A single wrap of the rope around an object. A round turn (pictured) is where the object is completely encircled.

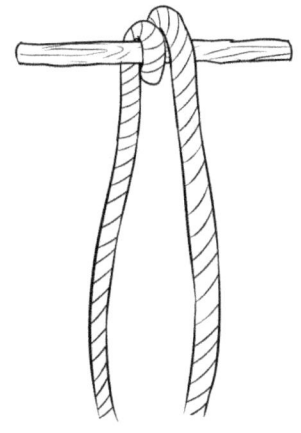

10 USEFUL KNOTS

Overhand Knot

This is the simplest of knots and is the basis of many other knots. An overhand knot is difficult to untie once it's tightened.

Make an underhand loop by taking the running end of the rope and passing it under the standing end. Pass the running end though the loop from the front to the back.

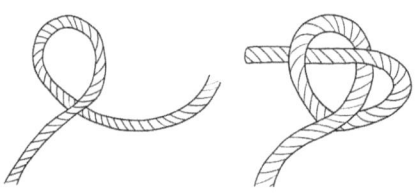

Pull both ends to tighten it.

The overhand knot can be made bulkier by passing the running end through the loop more times. Push the first turn into the middle of the knot.

Doing it twice makes a double overhand, and doing it three or more times creates a blood knot.

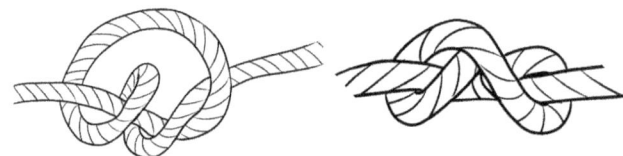

Bowline

A bowline is a fixed loop that will neither tighten nor slip under strain. It is good to tie around things you want to secure/tether, such as a raft or a person.

Hold the rope in your right hand, with the standing end at the rear. Make an overhand loop so that the loop faces to the left. Pass the running end up through the loop you made and then around the back of standing end.

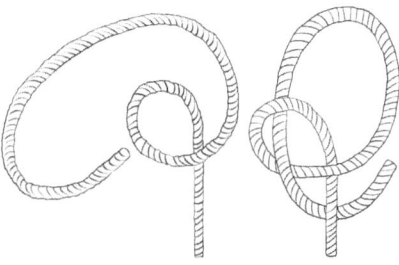

The running end then goes over the crossing point and back through the original loop.

To tighten the knot, pull the standing end and the doubled-up running end in opposite directions.

You can finish the bowline off with a stopper (overhand) knot tied against the side of the loop.

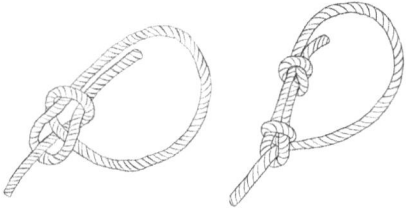

Once you can tie the bowline, practice doing it around things. It changes the orientation, so practice is needed.

Butterfly Loop

The butterfly loop (a.k.a. alpine butterfly or lineman's loop) is useful for creating a fixed loop in the middle of a rope. It's secure, can be loaded safely in multiple directions, and remains relatively easy to untie even after a heavy load.

Among other things, the butterfly loop is a very good knot to use to shorten a rope or to exclude a damaged section. Doing so is preferable to cutting a rope, since a rejoined rope has less strength.

Get a bight of the rope and twist it twice in the same direction, so you have two crossing points and therefore two loops.

For ease of explanation, the loop furthest away from the ends of the rope will be loop one, and the loop between the ends of the rope and loop one will be called loop two.

Grab the tip of the bight of loop one and bring it beyond the crossing point of loop two.

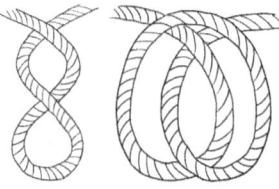

Next, bring the tip of loop one up through loop two.

Pull all ends to tighten.

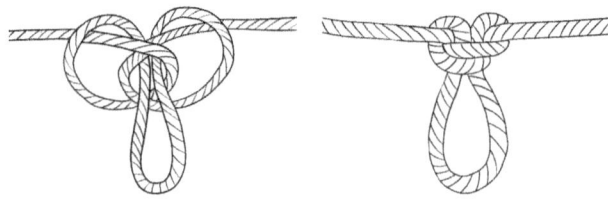

Cow Hitch

The cow hitch (a.k.a. lark's head) is not a very secure knot, but it is quick to tie and useful when making nets and other rope constructions.

To ensure it doesn't work itself loose, equal strain must be applied to both ends. Create a bight in the rope by doubling it up.

Pass this bight around the object you want to tie onto. Pull both ends of the rope through the bight you created, and then pull them both tight.

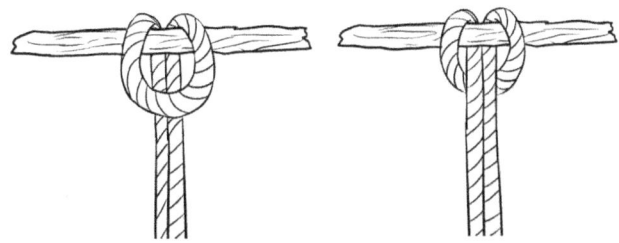

Cow hitch with toggle. This variation is useful when the two ends are secured and only the bight can be passed around the object.

Pass the bight around the object and then put a toggle between the bight and the standing ends to secure it in place.

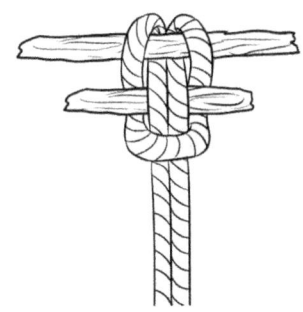

Figure-Eight

A figure-eight knot can do all the same things as the overhand knot, but is much easier to untie.

Make an upwards-facing overhand loop, and then make the running end pass back under the standing end. Pass the running end back through the first loop you made.

Pull both ends away from each other to tighten the knot.

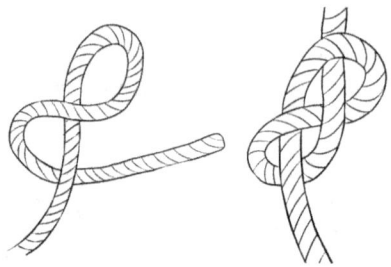

Figure-Eight Bend

The figure-eight bend is a fairly easy and secure way to join two ropes together. It's also good for making a prusik loop of rope, which can be used for ascending. It's best done with ropes of equal width, especially if it will hold a critical load.

Tie a loose figure-eight in the end of one of the ropes. Follow the path of the original figure-eight with the other rope, much as you would with a threaded figure-eight). Ensure that there's no crossover in the rope and that the ends face in opposite directions. Pull on all ends to tighten them.

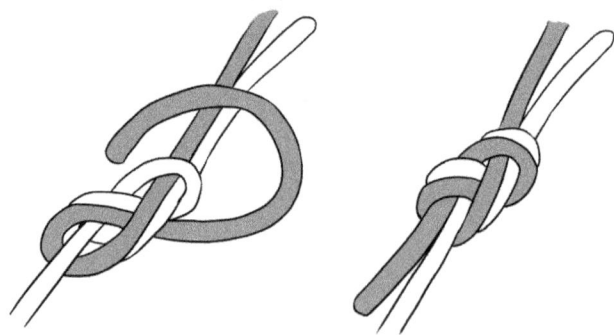

Half Hitch

The half hitch is easy to tie and easy to untie even after considerable load. It's designed to take load on the standing end.

Due to its simplicity, it's relatively easy to work loose. To prevent this, the half hitch is usually used in conjunction with other knots. Common examples are the round turn and two half hitches, which use three less secure knots to create one very secure knot that remains easy to tie and untie.

Some common uses for the half hitch on its own are as a backup knot and to use up any leftover rope so it's out of the way.

To tie the half hitch, loop the rope around the object. Bring the running end behind and then back over the standing end. The running end then threads through the loop above the crossing point created.

In this picture, the half hitch is loose, but in actual use it should be pulled tight and repeated (two half hitches) in order to create a more secure knot.

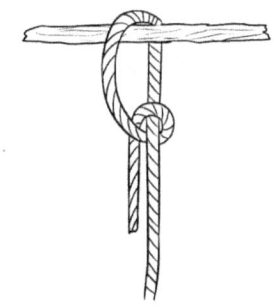

Reef Knot

A reef knot (a.k.a. square knot) is a good binding knot which is easy to tie and untie.

Many people may use the reef knot to join two ropes together. This is not advised, especially if the rope will be bearing load. There are far better joining knots, which are specifically designed for the job.

To tie a reef knot, put the rope around the object you want to bind. Take the left end, pass it over the right from the bottom, and then tuck it under the right end. Now take this new right end, cross it over the left end, and then tuck it under. Pull the left strands and the right strands apart to tighten the knot.

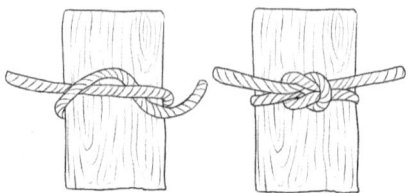

An easy way to remember this is with the formula "left over right and under, right over left and under."

Round Turn and Two Half Hitches

This knot is fast to tie and very secure. It's also fairly easy to untie, even when placed under heavy strain.

To create the round turn, loop the running end of the rope around your object so the rope completely encloses it.

Tie a half hitch by bringing the running end behind the standing end. Make a turn around the standing end, and then thread it through the gap you made between the running and standing ends.

Create a second half hitch in the same way, ensuring it's underneath the first half hitch. Pull both ends to tighten.

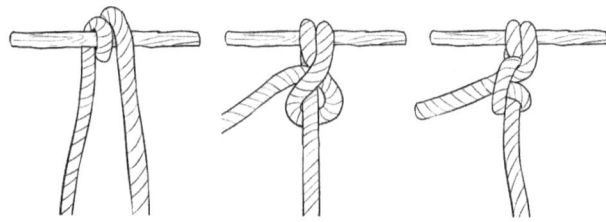

Surgeon's Knot

A variation of the reef knot is the surgeon's knot, which is more secure.

To tie a surgeon's knot, make an extra turn when tying the "left over right" part. This keeps the knot in place while you tie the rest of the knot. You could also make an extra turn in the "right over left" part to make it even more secure.

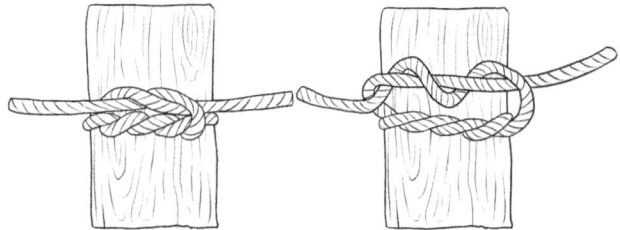

EMERGENCY ROPING

The methods described in this section make use of the knots previously described. These are techniques you may find useful in a survival situation.

Warning: The following techniques are reserved for "no other option" survival situations. If you choose to practice them, take all the necessary precautions to ensure your safety.

DESCENDING

The technique for rappelling with only a rope is known as the Dulfersitz method.

For this to work, you need a rope that's at least twice the length of the distance you wish to descend and that's strong enough to hold your weight.

Find the middle of the rope and wrap it around a solid anchor. Ensure it's not rubbing against any sharp edges and test its stability with all your weight. Jerk on it to make sure.

Pass both ends of the rope between your legs from front to back, and then to the left of your body, over your right shoulder, and down your back.

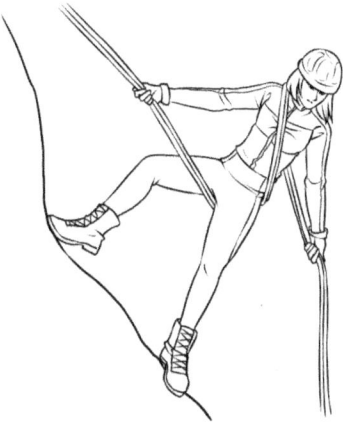

For comfort (and if you have the resources) you can put some padding around your shoulders and groin.

Hold the rope in front with your left hand and at the back with your right.

Plant your feet firmly against the slope about 45cm apart, and lean back so that the rope supports your weight. Do not try to hold yourself up with your hands.

Step slowly downwards while lowering your hands one at a time.

ASCENDING

Prusiking up a rope is a self-rescue method used by climbers. It's a relatively safe way to ascend a rope when there is no easy way to climb out. It can also be used in reverse if you need to descend.

Climbers will have proper equipment such as harnesses and carabineers, but chances are you will not. Still, prusiking up a rope without a harness is safer than trying to ascend without using a prusik system. Improvised harnesses, or even just a short rope tied around the waist using a bowline, can (and should) also be made if you have enough resources to do so.

The first thing you must do is create two closed loops. These will be your prusik loops. Many types of knots can be used to create a closed loop, but most of them are not safe to use when prusiking.

Climbers often use a double fisherman's knot, but a faster way is to use a figure-eight bend. This type of bend knot is also easier to tie than a double fisherman's and easier to untie, even after your weight has been on it.

Your two prusik loops should be made from rope about half the diameter of the rope you are going to ascend or descend. Ideally, one rope will be about 20cm longer than you are tall, and the second rope will be twice your height.

The rope you use for your prusik loops must strong enough to hold you if you fall. This doesn't just mean it can hold your weight; it has to be strong enough to handle the shock load.

Prusik Hitch

Once you've made your prusik loops, you'll use the prusik hitch to attach them to the rope you want to climb (the main line).

Put the loop across your main line, with the joining knot (figure-eight bend) facing the right. Wrap your prusik loop around the main line on the knotted side. Do this at least twice. The more wraps you make, the more friction you'll have.

Slowly tighten the loops As you do so, ensure all the lines are neatly next to each other. Do not let them overlap or cross each other. As you tighten the loops, do your best to position the figure-eight bend close to the main line.

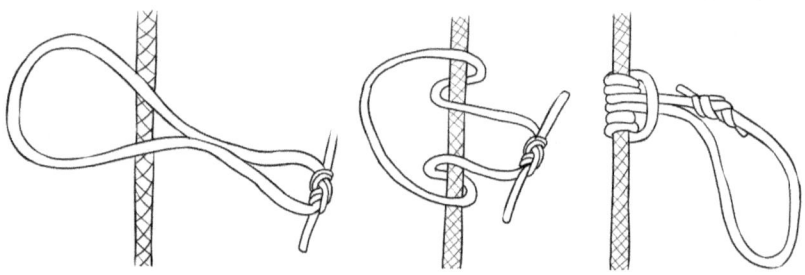

Ascending the Main Line Using Prusik Loops

Tie both prusik loops onto the main line using prusik hitches. Tie the smaller prusik loop above the larger one.

A prusik hitch works because you can slide it up, but it doesn't slip when downward tension is applied. Test it well with all your weight before using it to climb. Add extra turns if needed.

Attach the top prusik loop to your harness.

Note: Rope-on-rope friction can cut rope. If you have a carabiner, use it. If not, just be extra careful there's not too much friction between your harness and the prusik loop.

Slide the top prusik loop up as high as you can reach.

Slide the bottom prusik loop to about head height, or as high as you can get it and still put your foot in it. Put your foot in the loop and stand up. The joining knot of the prusik loop is the weak part, so keep off it.

Slide the top prusik loop as high as possible, and then put your weight on it by sitting in your harness. Now slide your bottom prusik loop up as high as possible and put your foot in it. Stand up and slide the top prusik loop up again. Repeat this motion.

To descend, just reverse the motions.

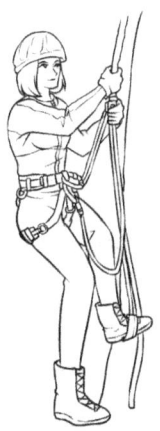

Ascending Without a Harness

It is possible to ascend using prusik loops with no harness, but doing so is extremely risky and uses considerably more energy. Sufficient strength is needed.

Make your loops smaller than usual and have at least two of them, preferably four.

Assuming you're using four prusik loops, the top two are for your hands and the bottom two are for your feet. You want them all to be fairly snug so you can slide them up with minimal movement.

Place your feet in the two bottom prusik loops and hold on to the top ones with your hands. Slide your hands up with the top prusik loops as high as you can. Pull yourself up and use your legs to slide the bottom prusik loops up as high as you can, then stand up while sliding the top prusik loops up again. Repeat this process.

Brake and Squat

If you don't have any rope to use as prusik loops, you can use the brake-and-squat method to climb the rope.

Let the rope fall to the outside of one of your legs. Step on the rope with the foot closest to it, then put your other foot underneath it. You're now in the basic position.

Grab the rope as high up as possible and hang off it. Bring your feet up as high as possible (pull yourself up and bring your knees to your chest) and place them in the basic position. This position locks the rope in so you can stand (and rest if needed). Reach up as high as you can again and repeat the process.

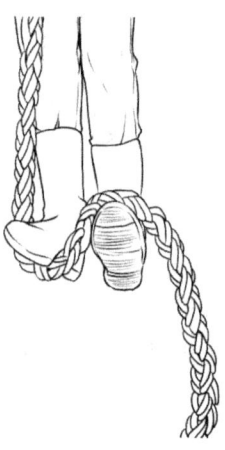

Ladder of Knots

A series of overhand knots tied at intervals along a smooth rope will make climbing much easier.

Rope Ladder

One way to make a rope ladder is to tie as many fixed loops (butterfly loops work well) in a rope as you need hand- and footholds.

Another way is by using two ropes (or one rope doubled up). Tie fixed loops opposite each other along the ropes. As you do so, put sticks (the rungs of the ladder) in the loops and slowly tighten the knot around them to hold them in place. Allow the rung ends to protrude out the sides of the knots a bit so they won't slip out.

Related Chapters:

- Improvised Harnesses

IMPROVISED HARNESSES

Improvised rope harnesses may not be that comfortable, but they are very useful to know how to make.

Triple Bowline

A triple bowline is basically a bowline made with a doubled-up line.

It produces three loops which can be used (among other things) as a sit sling or a lifting harness, with one loop around each thigh and the other around the chest.

Tie it in the exact same way as a bowline, using the middle of the rope. Do not use the ends. The running end must protrude out far enough to create the third loop.

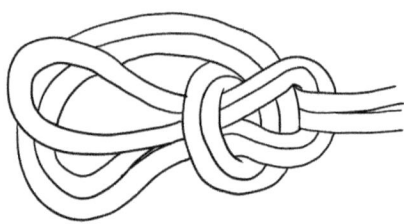

When using this to haul people, be careful of the pressure the rope may create on the chest. A foot loop can be made to release the pressure.

Swiss Seat

This is an improvised harness that's good enough to use when doing things such as using prusik loops for ascension, assuming you don't have a commercial harness.

Find the center of the rope. Loop it around your waist and tie the first half of a surgeon's knot at your front.

Pass the ends between your legs and then tuck them up through the wrap you made around your waist, on either side of your waist.

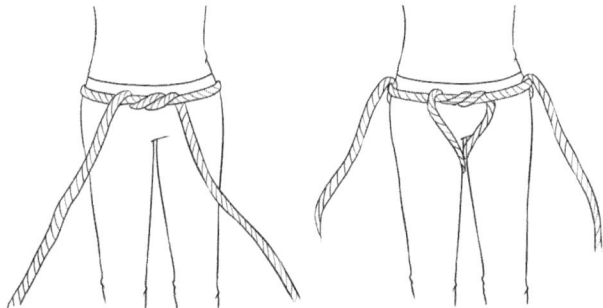

Pull down on the ends as you do a few squats. This will tighten it as well as check for comfort. Next, do a full wrap around your "belt" with each end of the rope.

Tie the ends together using a reef knot. Do it a little off center to make room for a carabiner. Make half hitches with the leftover rope that goes around both "belts."

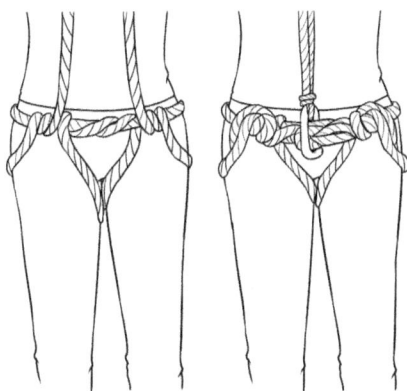

SELF-RESCUE BOWLINE

The self-rescue bowline is good to learn in case you find yourself in a "man overboard" situation or something similar. It is tying a bowline around your waist with only one hand.

Wrap the rope around your waist so that both the standing and running ends are to your front, with your body (waist) between them. In this demonstration, the running end is on your right.

Hold the running end in your right, hand allowing at least 15cm of rope beyond your hand.

Without letting go of the running end, bring it over the standing part to make a crossing point.

Bring it up though the gap created between your body and the crossing point. The rope will be wrapped around your hand.

Using your fingers, but without letting go of the rope, pass the running end under the standing part, just beyond the first crossing point. This creates a second crossing point.

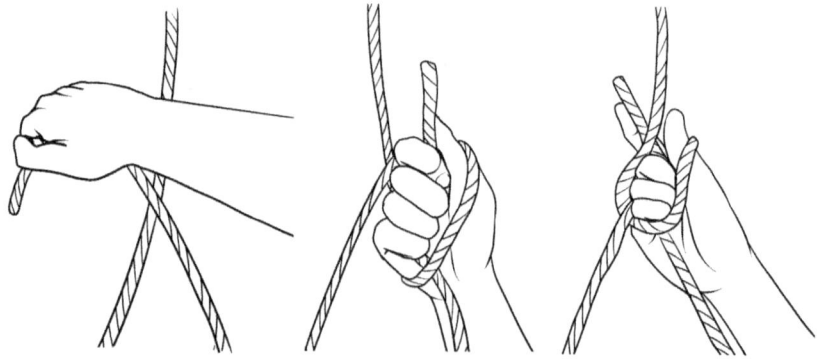

Continue to maneuver the running end with your fingers so that it feeds between the two crossing points. It feeds from the top down. You should end up holding the running end.

Once that's accomplished, pull your hand out from the loop on your wrist, bringing the running end with you. Pull the knot tight.

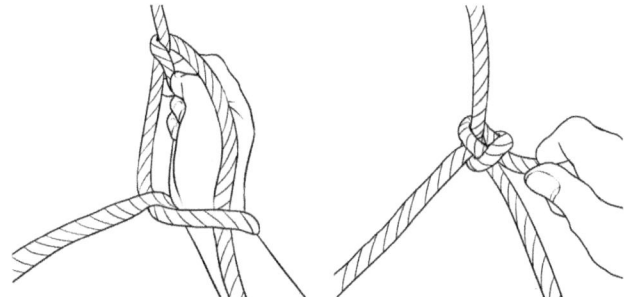

RIVER CROSSING WITH ROPE

In a survival situation, crossing a river can be an extremely risky venture. Using this method will reduce a lot of the risk, although it will still be dangerous.

You need at least three people and a rope three times the width of the river.

The first and last people to cross should be the strongest in the group, with the stronger of the two going first.

Tie the rope into a large loop and secure the person who is going to cross first (person A) to the loop. Tie a butterfly loop in the rope and put it over his/her chest.

As person A crosses, the other two let the rope out as needed. They must do their best to keep the rope out of the water, and be ready to haul person A back if needed.

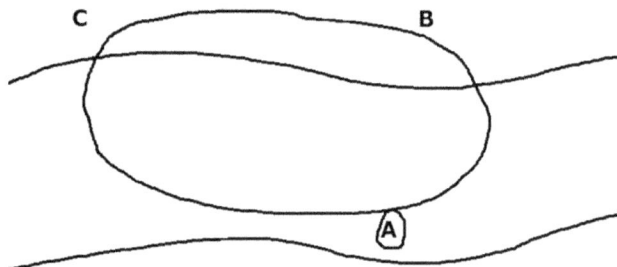

Person A is the only one secured to the rope.

When person A reaches the other side, he/she unties him-/herself.

As many people as needed can now cross (B), one at a time, by securing themselves to the rope and crossing over.

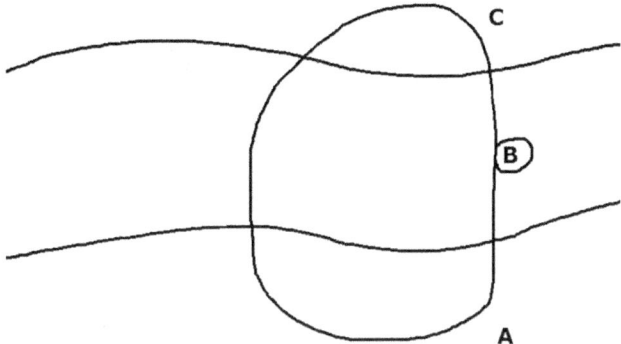

Although multiple people can help while others are crossing, the strongest person (A) should take most of the strain by being as close to directly across from the person crossing as possible.

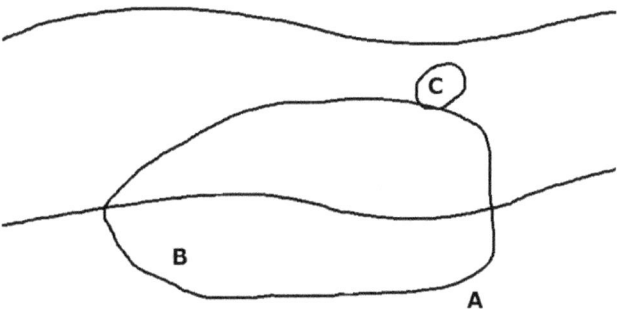

MAKING A GILL NET

A gill net is time- and resource-intensive to construct, but is very effective at catching marine life or birds when you're in a survival situation.

Tie a suspension line between two trees for you to work off. Get many lengths of cord and tie them to the suspension line using cow hitches. Space them about 10cm apart. Tie the separate lines together using overhand knots. Space them vertically, about 10cm apart.

Another line can be tied between the trees as a guideline. Use the guideline to ensure you tie the joining overhand knots at the same height.

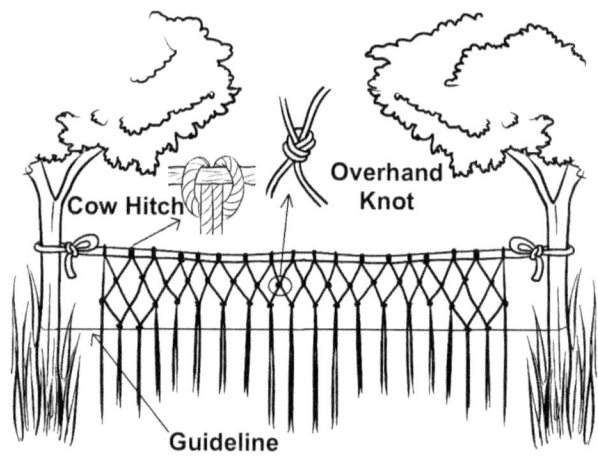

Once you're finished, you can attach floats at the top and weights at the bottom. This will keep the net vertical in the water.

Stretch the gill net across a river. It will be most effective in still water, such as a lake (near the inlet and outlet are good locations) or in the backwater of a large stream.

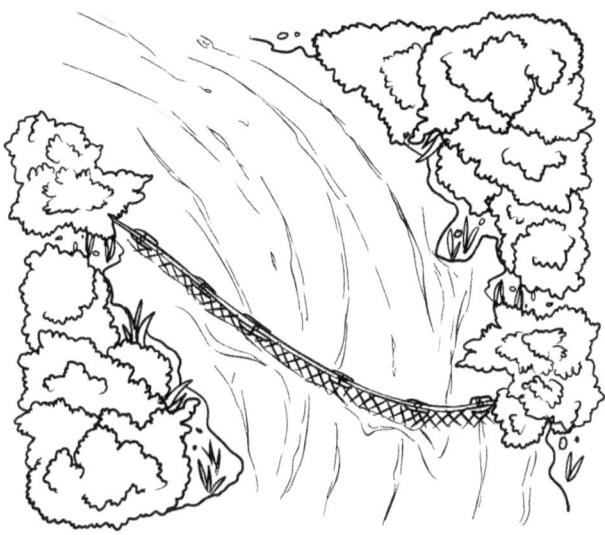

The gill net will catch everything, so don't deploy it for very long.

When in the open sea, pass a gill net under the keel of your raft or boat from end to end. It will catch whatever is attracted to the shelter created by your craft.

MAKING ROPE

Rope (cord, string, etc.) is extremely useful and can be improvised from many different materials, including fabric, fishing line, and shoelaces.

When there is no such thing available (or you're not willing to sacrifice it), then other common materials can be made into rope. Suitable ones include:

- Animal hair.
- Inner bark (cedar, chestnut, elm, hickory, linden, mulberry, and white oak work well). Shred the plant fibers from the inner bark.
- Fibrous stems (honeysuckle and stinging nettles work well).
- Grasses.
- Palms.
- Rushes.
- Sinew (dry tendons of large game).
- Rawhide.
- Vines (strong vines can be used without any other preparation, but plant fibers spun together will be more durable).

Making Rope from Plant Material

When you think you have a suitable plant material, see if it can withstand the following tests.

Note: Stiff fibers can be softened by steaming them or soaking them in water.

- Pull the ends in opposite directions.
- Twist and roll it between your fingers.
- Tie an overhand knot in it.

To turn the material into rope, twine it together. Collect a small pile of it. Divide it in half and rotate one half before recombining them. This ensures an even consistency in your rope.

Get a bunch of the material, depending on how thick you want your cordage/rope, and knot it together at one end.

Divide the remaining side of the bundle into two even sections and twist them both clockwise to create two strands.

Next, twist one of the strands around the other counterclockwise. Tie the end to prevent it from unraveling.

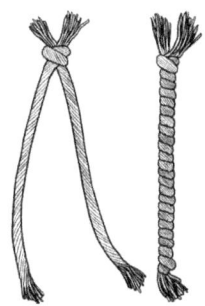

You can join shorter lengths together by splicing them. Do so by twisting the ends of their strands together while they're still in two lengths, before the counterclockwise twisting. Twist one small bunch on each side (for each of the strands) and then just continue to twist as before. You can do this as much as you want until you get the desired length of rope.

Thicker ropes can be made by using larger bundles of grass or by twisting multiple ropes together.

Making Rope from Animals

In a survival situation, you may be fortunate enough to capture game. Waste nothing.

Sinew is an excellent material for small lashings. Remove the tendons from game animals and dry them. Once they're completely dry, hammer them until they are fibrous. Add some moisture so you can twist the fibers together. You could also braid them together, which would make a stronger product.

Sinew is sticky when wet and hardens when dry. You can lash small items together while the sinew is wet, and since it dries hard, the actual use of knots is not necessary.

When the job is too big for sinew, rawhide can be used. Skin any medium to large game and clean the skin very well. Make sure there's no fat or meat, though hair/fur is okay. Dry it completely. If there are folds that will capture moisture, you'll need to stretch the skin out. Once it's dry, cut it into a continuous 5mm- to 10mm-wide length. The best way to do this is to begin in the middle of the skin and cut outwards in circles, expanding the spiral as you go.

To use the rawhide, soak it until it's soft. This usually takes two to four hours. Use it wet and stretch it as much as you can as you do so. Leave to dry.

THROWING ROPE

Knowing how to throw rope properly will greatly increase the distance you can throw it. In most cases, you should aim to throw it further than you think you need to. If you intend to keep one end of the rope (which is usually the case), be sure to secure it to something.

Note: Even when throwing all the rope to someone, it's a good idea to secure one end. If your throw doesn't clear the obstacle, you can pull the rope back, and if it does, you can just untie the rope and your friend can pull it over.

Tie a weight or several overhand knots to the end you're going to throw over. Coil half the rope in the palm of your right hand. Coil the rest of it on your fingers.

Stand on one end to secure it, or tie it to something. Grab the coils you made on your fingers with your left hand.

As you throw, release the right-hand coils a split second before the left. When throwing a weighted rope over a branch, beware of it swinging back.

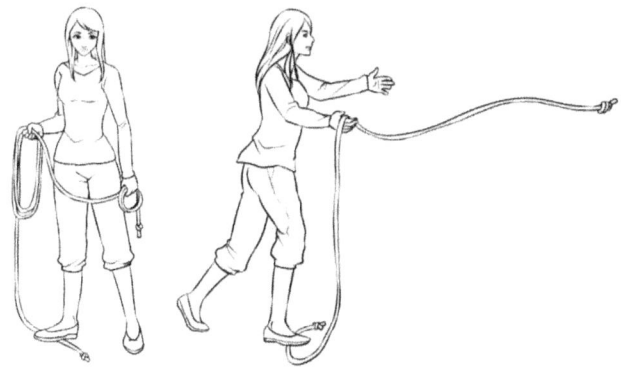

BOULDERING

Bouldering is the act of climbing without the use of ropes and harnesses.

I haven't met many people who didn't enjoy climbing when they were a child. Trees, rocks, the roof of the family home—I loved to climb them all, and perhaps you did too. The point is that as children, we needed no instruction on how to climb; we just did. That's because climbing is a natural instinct in all of us.

As we get older and stop "practicing," we lose the skills. Luckily, they can be relearned, and in the process we can also learn the best methods to use.

The only intention of this section is to introduce the basic maneuvers and foundational techniques needed for bouldering. The basics are all you really need. Learn and practice them.

Safety note: When bouldering, NEVER climb higher than you would be willing to jump down. It's also wise to use a crash mat.

SAFETY TAP

When you're bouldering, there will be many times when you'll need to drop down to the ground. In these cases, a technique borrowed from parkour, called the safety tap, is useful in preventing injury.

The following is an excerpt from the book *Essential Parkour Training* by Sam Fury.

www.SFNonfictionBooks.com/Essential-Parkour

Using the safety tap allows you to cushion your landing. It's good for those times when rolling may not be possible, such as when there's a lack of room, although it's best to use rolls when dropping from greater heights and/or on angles.

To do the safety tap, drop down from a ledge. Start with small drops and work your way up as your confidence builds.

Land on the balls of both feet at the same time, and then roll your heels down towards the ground.

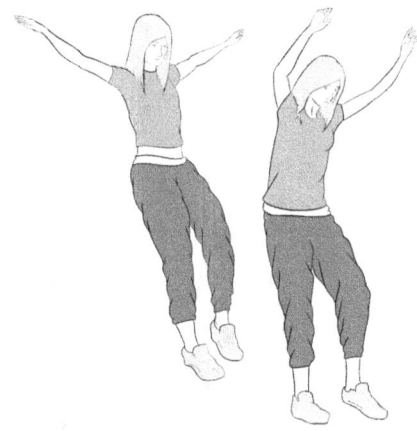

Bend your knees as you land to absorb the shock. Depending on the impact, you can go all the way into a crouch.

Don't slam your wrists down. They are used for assistance and/or balance, but should not be sustaining any major impact.

Spring back up, using the momentum to continue your run.

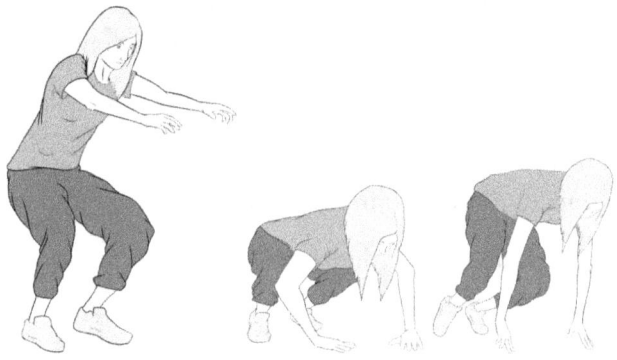

Try to land as softly and quietly as possible. This is true with most things in parkour. The quieter you are, the softer you are, which means you put less pressure on your joints. Since the practical use for parkour is to run from your enemy, it's advantageous to be as silent as possible.

When dropping down from a wall, it's a good idea to turn away from the obstacle. You may have to use your feet to push away from the wall a little so you can get the room to turn.

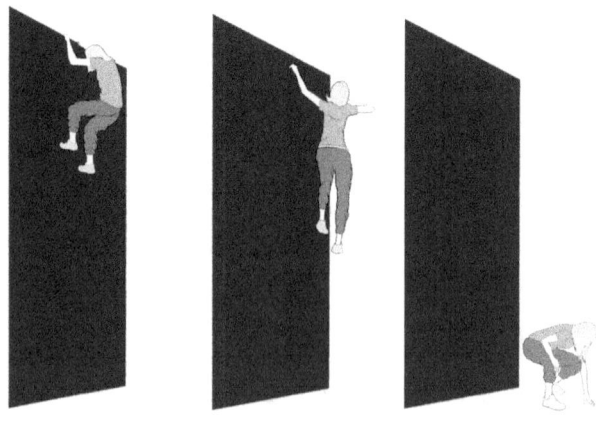

BASIC PRINCIPLES

Holds are what you place your feet and hands on when climbing. They are what you "hold" on to.

Climb with Your Legs

Your legs are your main climbing tool. Your arms are primarily for keeping balance. Be sure to:

- Move your feet up the wall first and use your legs to push you up.
- Know where you will place your foot before moving it.
- Place your foot carefully and firmly.
- Use the edges of your feet or the ball of your big toe.
- Press your foot firmly downwards and into the wall.
- Trust that you can stand.

Plan Your Route

Plan your route before you start climbing and at least one move ahead while you're climbing. Adjust your plan as needed as you do.

Climb Smoothly

Remember to:

- Climb smoothly and fluidly. Don't pause between moves.
- Step lightly, and only reach as much as needed to grab the hold.
- Grip only as hard as you need to.
- Breathe.

Gaining Reach

There are several ways to increase your reach.

One way is to turn away from a hold and reach backwards for it. This is similar to reaching for something far under a bed.

Another method is to stand straight. Keep your hips close to the wall with your weight over your feet, as opposed to leaning against the rock.

Your last choice is bumping. This is where you gain momentum off one hold in order to reach a better one.

HOLDS AND GRIPS

Edges

An edge is a horizontal hold with a part you can grab onto. It's often flat, but sometimes has a lip you can pull on.

Crimp Grip

Crimping is grabbing the edge with your fingertips flat and your fingers arched above the tips. Crimping too hard can cause tendon damage.

Full Crimp

To do the full crimp**,** place the pads of your fingertips on an edge and curl your fingers so that the second joint is sharply flexed. Press your thumb on top of your index finger's fingernail to secure the grip.

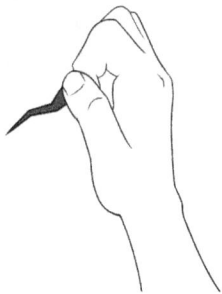

Half Crimp

If you let your thumb press against the side of your index finger, you are using the half crimp.

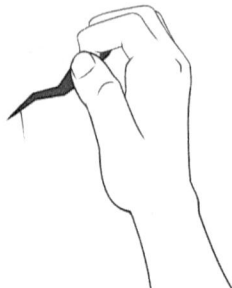

The half crimp is weaker, but less damaging to your fingers. If you have the option, use the half crimp.

Slopers

Slopers are rounded handholds without an edge. They're easiest to grab if they are above you. Keep your arms straight for maximum leverage when gripping them.

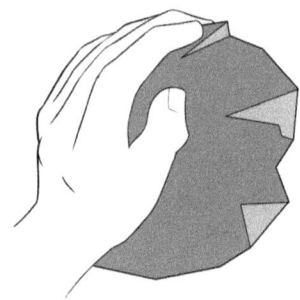

Open-hand Grip

To grab a sloper, use the open-hand grip.

Use the friction of your skin against the rock surface. Feel around with your fingers to find grip spots. Wrap your hand onto the hold, with your fingers close together, and then feel around with your thumb to see if there's a bump you can press against.

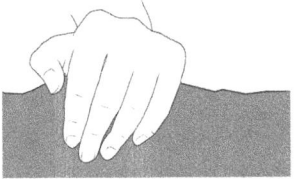

Pinches

Pinches are holds which can be gripped by pinching them with your fingers on one side and your thumb on the other.

If a pinch hold is small, use your thumb opposed to your index finger, with your middle finger stacked on top. With larger pinch holds, oppose your thumb with all your fingers.

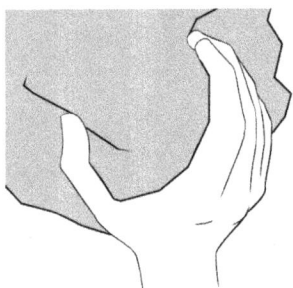

Side Pulls

Side pulls are holds that you pull sideways instead of straight down, due to their orientation. You can pull outward on the side pull while pushing a foot in the opposite direction to keep you in place.

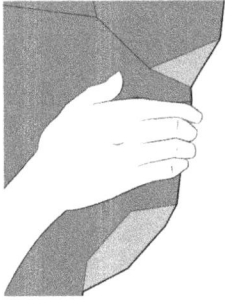

Pockets

Pockets are holes in the rock surface which you can place your finger(s) in.

Insert as many fingers as you can comfortably fit into a pocket. Use your strongest fingers first. Feel inside the pocket to find a surface you can pull against.

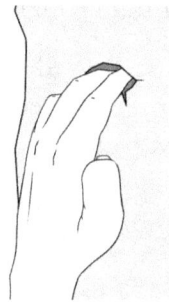

Gastons

A gaston is a hold oriented either vertically or diagonally, and is usually to your front.

Grab it with your fingers and palm facing into the rock and your thumb pointing downward. Bend your elbow at a sharp angle and point it away from your body. Crimp your fingers on the edge and pull outward.

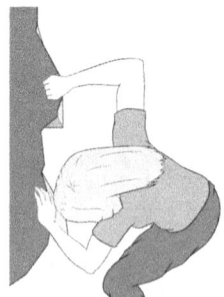

Undercling

An undercling is any hold that's gripped on its underside. It requires body tension and opposition.

Grip the rock with your palm facing up and your thumb pointing out. Pull out on the undercling and push your feet against the wall.

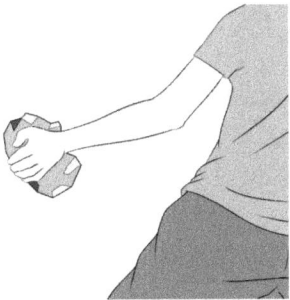

Palming

If no handhold exists, keep your hand in place by pushing into a dimple in the rock with the heel of your palm.

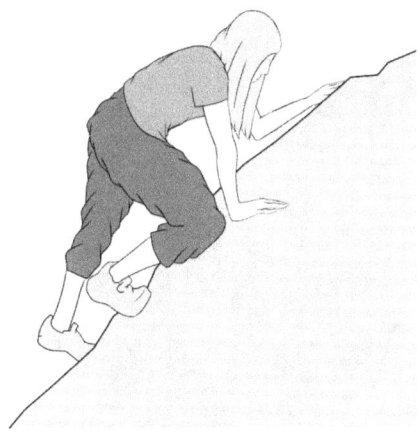

Matching Hands

Matching hands is when you place your hands next to each other on the same hold so you can change hands.

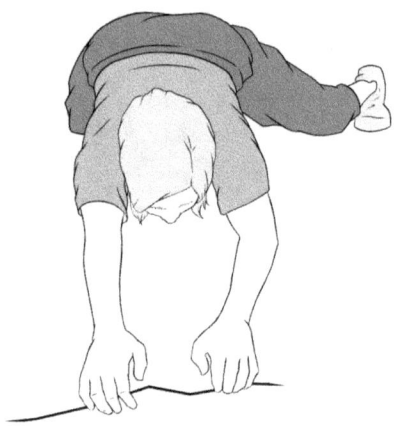

A similar technique can be done with your feet. Do so by slowly replacing one foot with the other and without jumping.

It can also be done with a hand and foot.

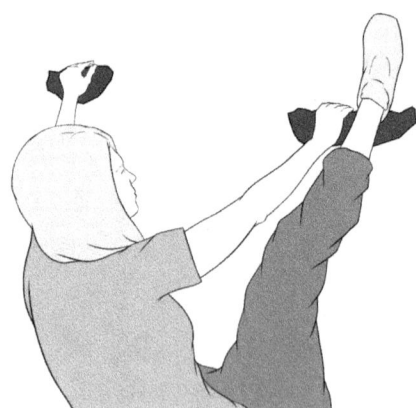

Plan ahead to minimize matching. For example, reach for an extra hold over so that your trailing hand can have its own hold.

FOOT TECHNIQUES

Smearing

To do this, push the flat of your foot hard on the wall, using friction to hold you up. If you want to go up, direct the force slightly downwards. Return to a foothold as soon as you can.

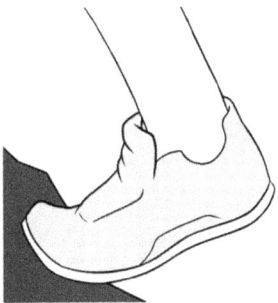

Back-stepping

To use this technique, step on a hold so that the outside of your hip faces into the rock, allowing for longer reach in the same direction as the foot that you stepped back with.

For an exaggerated back-step, drop one knee toward the ground with the other pointing up.

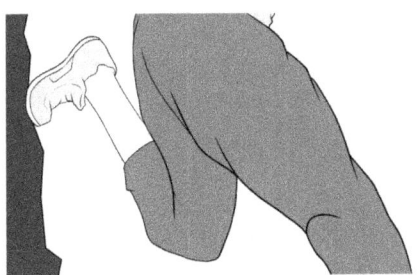

Flagging

Flagging is used to balance your body when reaching for a hold. Cross one foot behind the other to avoid swinging out from the rock.

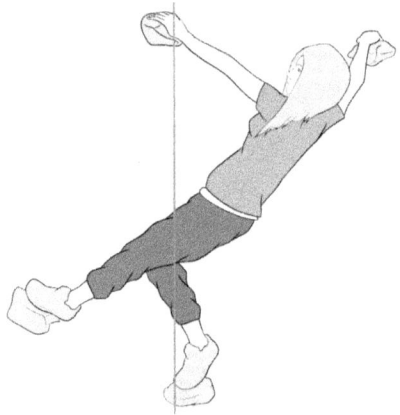

Stemming

Stemming is used to climb opposing walls, otherwise known as chimneys. Press a foot into one of the walls and your other foot against the other. Push out with opposing force to hold your weight up, and do the same with your hands.

Hold your weight with your arms/hands and shift both feet up. Once you have a good grip with your feet, hold your weight with your legs and move your hands up. Repeat this "shuffling" with your hands and feet to climb the chimney.

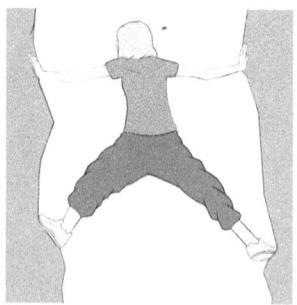

Hooking

Heel and toe hooks can aid in balance and provide leverage for movement.

There are a few ways to use a hook. For example, you can make one with your foot to climb onto a ledge.

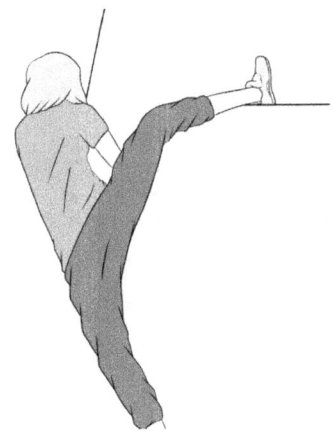

Hook under a rock to maintain your stability while you're negotiating an overhang.

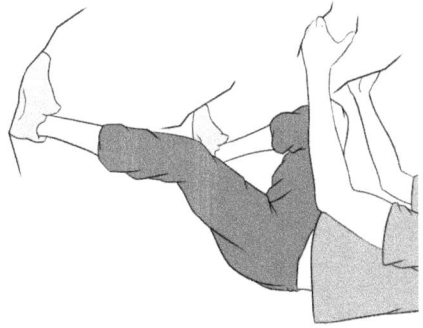

MANTLE

Use the mantle to climb up onto a ledge.

Get up close to the ledge. Pull yourself up, rock sideways, turn your hand around, and push yourself up until you can place a foot and stand up.

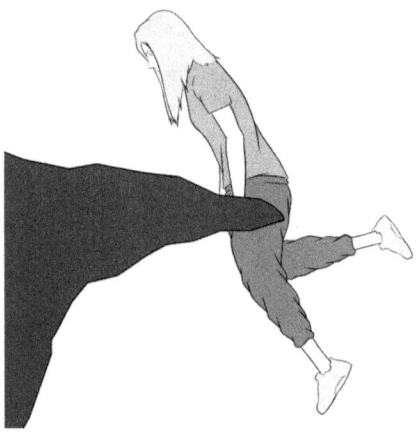

Exercises such as pulls-ups and muscle-ups will help build the strength needed to do mantles.

Pull-Ups

Pull-ups are an excellent all-body exercise, and doing them regularly will help condition you for wall climb-ups and eventually the muscle-up.

Grab the bar with a grip slightly wider than shoulder width apart and with your palms facing away from you. Let yourself hang all the way down.

Pull yourself up by pulling your shoulder blades down and together. Keep your chest up and pull up until your chin is above the bar. Touch your chest to it.

As you're pulling up, keep your body in a vertical line. Do not swing. Concentrate on isolating your back and biceps. Pause at the top, and then lower yourself back down into the hanging position.

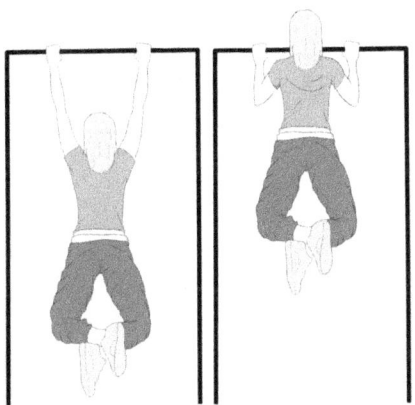

Muscle-Ups

Muscle-ups are used to get on top of higher obstacles when a wall climb-up cannot be used, such as with an overhanging ledge.

For both technique and conditioning reasons, you'll need to be proficient at the wall climb-up before attempting the muscle-up. The muscle-up is quite a physically demanding exercise. Progressing gradually is the key to success.

Start with the hanging knee-to-elbow raise. Hang off the bar and pull yourself up slightly to retract your shoulder blades. This helps keep you stable while you're doing the exercise.

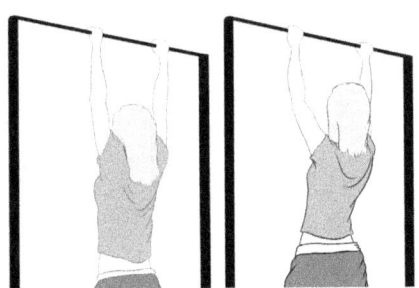

Keep your core tight and swing forward a little bit. As your body starts to swing back, thrust your knees to your chest.

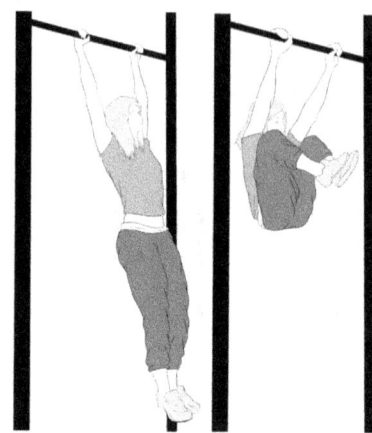

Next, you need to learn how to use the momentum from the hanging knee-to-elbow raise to pull yourself over the bar.

Start the raise as normal. At the height of your backswing, pull yourself forward and thrust your knees to your chest while allowing your wrists to rotate over the bar.

It will help if you have access to a lower bar to practice the movement. If not, then just keep it in mind when doing the muscle-up.

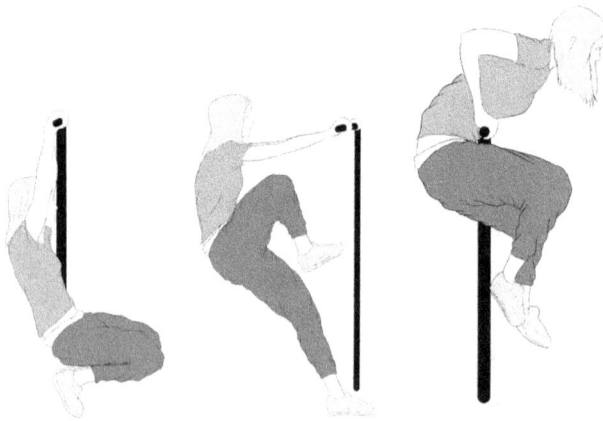

Now you can put everything together to do the muscle-up. It is important to use everything learnt so far. Remember to keep your core tight.

In addition to retracting your shoulder blades, pull your arms forward a little bit when pulling yourself over the bar.

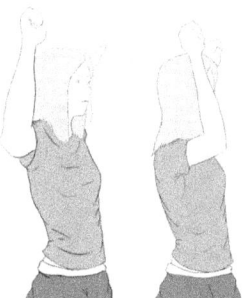

You can use some chalk to get extra grip, although you probably won't have this luxury in real-life scenarios.

Get some momentum and then thrust your knees to your chest.

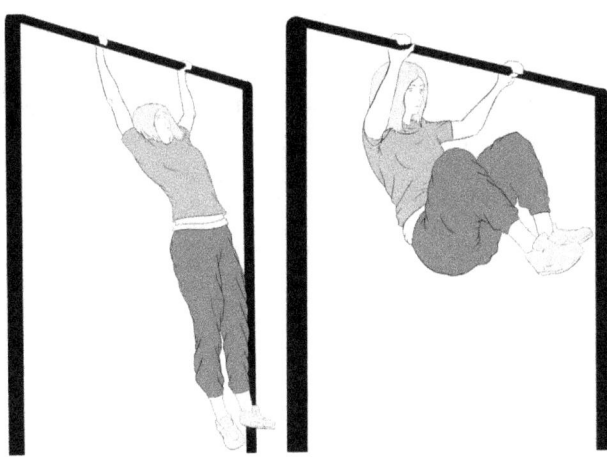

As you do so, ensure your wrists are loosened, and then at the right moment pull yourself up over the bar. Push yourself up until your arms are fully extended.

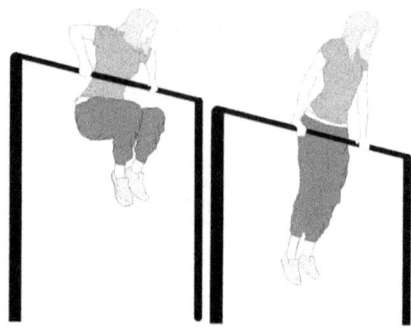

If this was an obstacle, you would bring your foot up and stand, just like in the wall-climb.

If you want to do multiple muscle-ups, you can use the momentum you gain when lowering yourself down to go into the next repetition.

Once you have built more strength, try to do the muscle-up with less and less swing, until you can do it from a dead hang.

You will also need to practice doing muscle-ups over hanging ledges, where there is no wall for your feet to push against. To do this, you need to adjust your technique a little, since you don't have a bar for your wrist to rotate over. Use the "pop" hand movement you use when doing a wall climb-up.

TYPES OF FACES

Slabs

A slab is any rock face than is angled at less than 90°.

To climb one, keep your weight centered on your feet. Stand upright on the rock and away from the slab surface.

Make small steps on small footholds rather than big steps on big holds. Plan the next three to five of your intended footholds ahead at a time. Aim for big holds and rest when you reach them.

As you climb, look for variations in the surface and smear on tiny holds.

Be precise with your toe placement. Feel the hold with a finger to find the best spot for your foot placement.

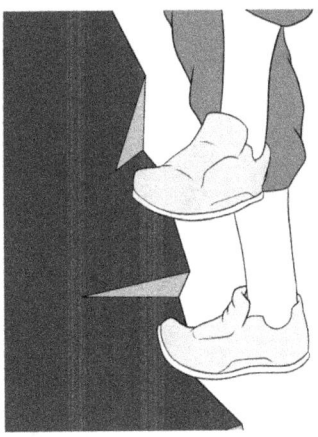

Vertical

Vertical faces are angled at 90°—that is, straight up (or close to it).

To climb one, keep your weight over your feet as much as possible. Use an upright body position, and use your hands and arms to pull if needed.

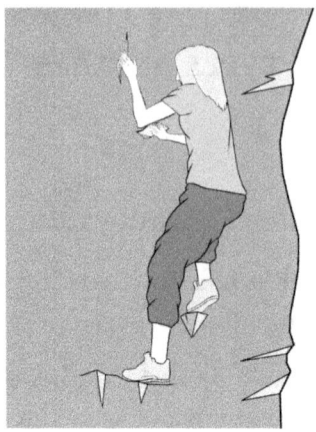

Overhangs

Overhangs are rock faces that are overhung or angled more than 90°.

When you're climbing them, heel and toe hooks are useful to take the weight off your arms.

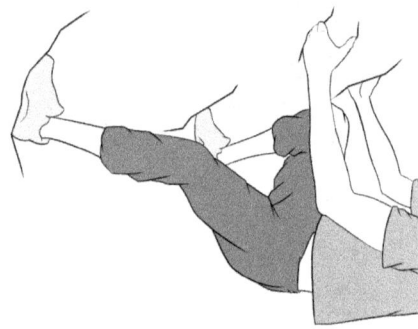

CRACK CLIMBING

Climb the natural cracks in the rock by jamming. Jamming is wedging your body parts into a crack. Doing so can cut your hands. Prevent this by taping your hands for protection.

Hand Jam

Wedge the side of your hand in the crack, with your thumb on top. Tuck your thumb into the palm of your hand.

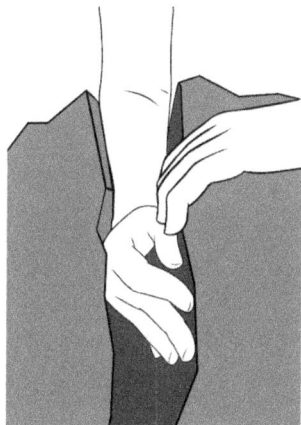

Expand your hand to exert opposing pressure against the walls of the crack. Hang your weight off your wedged hand.

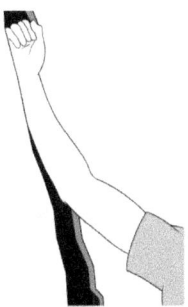

Foot Jam

Once your hands are jammed into the crack, lift a foot and push the front part of your shoe into the crack. Stand up on the jammed foot. Step the other foot up to calf level and jam it in the crack too.

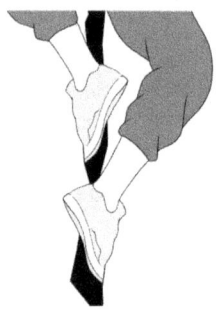

Shuffling

Move upward by shuffling your hands up the crack. There are three ways to do this:

- Move your top hand up first, then the lower one below it.
- Lift the bottom hand out of the crack and hand jam above your upper hand.
- Use the above two techniques together.

Do the same with your feet.

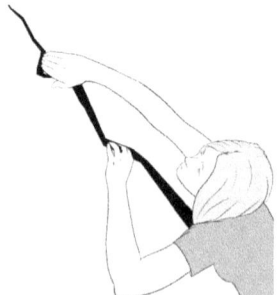

THANKS FOR READING

Dear reader,

Thank you for reading *Emergency Roping And Bouldering*.

If you enjoyed this book, please leave a review where you bought it. It helps more than most people think.

Don't forget your FREE book chapters!

You will also be among the first to know of FREE review copies, discount offers, bonus content, and more.

Go to:

https://offers.SFNonfictionBooks.com/Free-Chapters

Thanks again for your support.

REFERENCES

Auerbach, P. Constance, B Freer, L. (2018). *Field Guide to Wilderness Medicine.* Elsevier.

Beal, P. (2011). *Bouldering: Movement, Tactics, and Problem Solving (Mountaineers Outdoor Expert).* Mountaineers Books.

Brayak, D. Keenan, T. (2007). *Coopers Rock Bouldering Guide (Bouldering Series).* Falcon Guides.

Budworth, G. Dalton, J. (2016). *The Little Book of Incredibly Useful Knots: 200 Practical Knots for Sailors, Climbers, Campers & Other Adventurers.* Skyhorse.

Emerson, C. (2016). *100 Deadly Skills: Survival Edition.* Atria Books.

Hanson, J. (2015). *Spy Secrets That Can Save Your Life.* TarcherPerigee.

Hanson, J. (2018). *Survive Like a Spy.* TarcherPerigee.

Jarmin, C. (2013). *The Knot Tying Bible: Climbing, Camping, Sailing, Fishing, Everyday.* Firefly Books.

Jäger, J. Sundsten, B. (2014). *My First Book of Knots: A Beginner's Picture Guide (180 color illustrations).* Sky Pony.

Terrill, B. Dierkers, G. (2005). *The Unofficial MacGyver How-To Handbook.* American International Press.

Wiseman, J. (2015). *SAS Survival Guide.* William Collins.

AUTHOR RECOMMENDATIONS

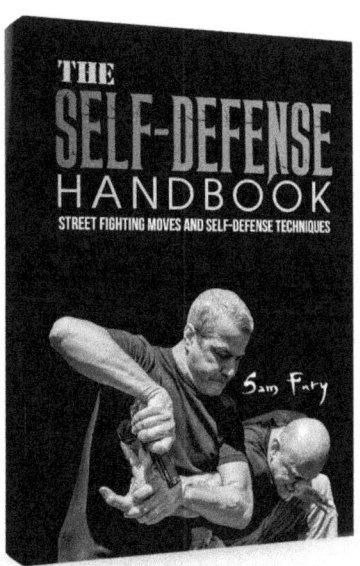

Teach Yourself Self-Defense

This is the only self-defense training manual you need, because these are the best street fighting moves around.

Get it now.

www.SFNonfictionBooks.com/Self-Defense-Handbook

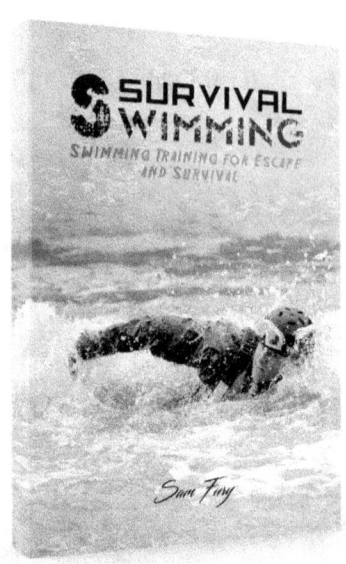

These Swimming Skills Will Save Your Life!

Teach yourself everything you need to survive in the water, because this is swim training for escape and survival..

Get it now.

www.SFNonfictionBooks.com/Survival-Swimming

ABOUT SAM FURY

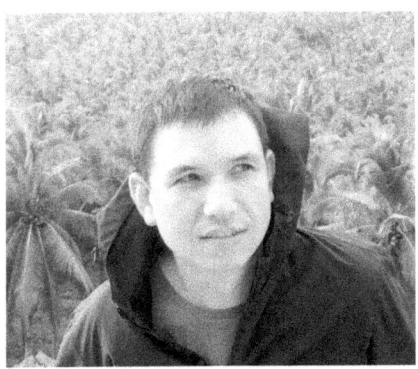

Sam Fury has had a passion for survival, evasion, resistance, and escape (SERE) training since he was a young boy growing up in Australia.

This led him to years of training and career experience in related subjects, including martial arts, military training, survival skills, outdoor sports, and sustainable living.

These days, Sam spends his time refining existing skills, gaining new skills, and sharing what he learns via the Survival Fitness Plan website.

www.SurvivalFitnessPlan.com

- amazon.com/author/samfury
- goodreads.com/SamFury
- facebook.com/AuthorSamFury
- instagram.com/AuthorSamFury
- youtube.com/SurvivalFitnessPlan

www.ingramcontent.com/pod-product-compliance
Lightning Source LLC
Chambersburg PA
CBHW071031080526
44587CB00015B/2574